The 'Permanent Weight Loss' Diet

How To Lose Weight Fast, Keep it Off & Renew
The Mind, Body & Spirit Through Fasting,
Smart Eating & Practical Spirituality - Volume 1

ROBERT DAVE JOHNSTON

Published by:

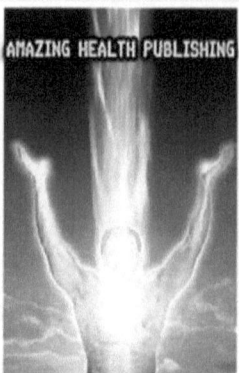

If you are interested in reading the next volume, follow Rob on Twitter @RobDaveJohnston

Copyright

Disclaimer & Legal Notices

The health-related information and suggestions contained in any of the books or written material mentioned above are based on the research, experience and opinions of the Author and other contributors. Nothing herein should be misinterpreted as actual medical advice, such as one would obtain from a Physician, or as advice for self-diagnosis or as any manner of prescription for self-treatment.

Neither is any information herein to be considered a particular or general cure for any ailment, disease or other health issue. The material contained within is offered strictly and solely for the purpose of providing Holistic health education to the general public. Persons with any health condition should consult a medical professional before entering this or any fasting, weight loss, detoxification or health related program.

Even if you suffer from no known illness, we recommend that you seek medical advice before starting any fasting, weight loss and/or detoxification program, and before choosing to follow any advice given this book. For any products or services mentioned or suggested in this book, you should read all packaging and instructions, as no substance, natural or drug, can be guaranteed to work in everyone.

Information and statements regarding dietary supplements, products or services mentioned in this book many not have been evaluated by the Food and Drug Administration and are not intended to diagnose, treat, cure, or prevent any disease. Never disregard or delay in seeking professional medical advice because of something you have read in this book.

Nothing that you read in this book should be regarded as medical or health advice. If you do anything recommended in this book, without the supervision of a licensed medical doctor, you do so at your own risk. Not recommended for persons with any health related condition unless supervised by a qualified health practitioner.

Because there is always some risk involved in any health-related program, the Author, Publisher and contributors assume no responsibility for any adverse effects or consequences resulting from the use of any suggested preparations or procedures described in any of the books or other written materials associated with the website FitnessThroughFasting.com. The author reserves the right to alter and update his opinions based on new conditions at any time.

Dedication

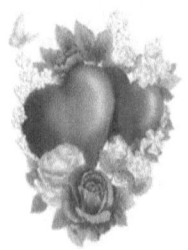

This series of books are dedicated to my mother Sonia Noemi, without whom I would not even be alive today. I love you mom. Thank you for never losing faith in me and supporting me, even when everything seemed hopeless and everyone else had given up on me. I owe you everything. I could collect all of the precious stones on this earth and lay them on your lap, and even still, I would not even come close to giving back to you all that you have given me.

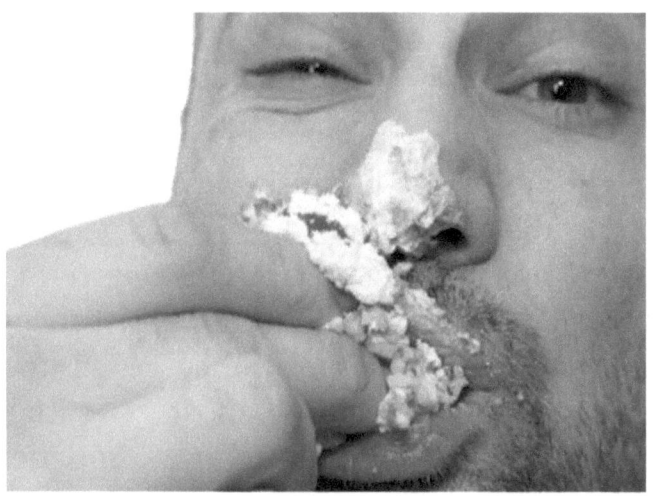

"Any time that I even tried (for just a few hours) to stop eating, I was wacked with intense physical and mental discomfort. My only option at the time was to give in... to get my fix."

Chapter 1
Lazy Gluttons

The reason why so many people try to lose weight and fail is because they <u>do not stick to the diet until the miracle happens</u>. It's that simple. There is nothing '*mysterious*' about it. Many start the weight loss process. Few hang in there until they reach their goals. Why? Because most of these individuals are lazy gluttons ... impatient and petulant. They want what they want, when they want it and, by the way, they want it NOW! Never mind that it took 25 years for Steve to get as fat as he is. He wants an 'easy' solution, or he will get angry and refuse to talk. He has enough information on diets and weight loss to write an entire encyclopedia. But he won't put it to practice because, "it is too hard ... too uncomfortable." And, Lord knows... all discomfort must be shunned at any cost, right?

These individuals simply do not understand the reality that "*weight loss entails going through some hunger and sacrifice.*" Or maybe they do understand it but refuse to accept it. What perhaps never crosses their minds is that, *"whatever temporary hunger or discomfort one goes through initially is NOTHING in comparison to the joy, health and HUGE sense of accomplishment that comes later."* Yes... these individuals are myopic and immature. They want the results, but they are unwilling to pay the price. This attitude is common among professional dieters. I come across them all of the time.

When losing the weight takes a bit longer or requires more sacrifice than initially anticipated, they throw a tantrum and give up. Then they'll tell you that they are still fat because the diet they were following *"sucks and doesn't work."* It's always the fault of something external to them. In which category would you place yourself? Do you realize, in your heart and mind, that the **ONLY** way to reach your weight loss goals is to walk directly through the hunger and discomfort? Or are you still looking for the easier, softer way? I always like to say that taking action and going through the discomfort of dieting and getting fit **IS** the easiest way. The other alternative is to evade the issue, continue to look for shortcuts and - in so doing - waste precious years of life being overweight and in less than optimum health. So, yes... I am here to help you *'get it over with once and for all.'* Let me be honest: I have said some things about laziness and gluttony that, to some, may seem harsh. But it is not. It is the truth. And the reason why I know this is because I was in the very same boat for many years. I was obese, miserable and desperate to lose weight. But I was also lazy, arrogant and impatient. I could start a diet with guns blazing. However, a few weeks later, I had moved on to something else because the weight *"didn't come off fast enough."* So I am not being insensitive when I say that many overweight people are lazy, petulant gluttons. I say it because I myself lived it and acted the very same way. What changed? Simple: **I got sick and tired of being sick and tired**. I became fed up with my **BS** and decided that I would do <u>whatever it took</u> to lose the weight. That is the essence of this book.

A Hopeless Basket Case

Put the past behind you. Whatever failures you may have experienced with weight loss, forget about them. Dust yourself off and join me with a clean slate. It is time to go the distance and do this. There is no more time to waste lamenting or feeling sorry for ourselves. Tell me: Are you tired of always starting a diet but never finishing it? Are you tired of being fat? If you are, then good... hang on to that feeling. We're going to need it. I am going to give you the plan and structure - the same structure that helped me to lose more than 100 pounds and overcome 20+ years of binge eating disorder. I **was a hopeless basket case that nobody wanted to deal with.** Everyone was waiting for me to eat myself to death or commit suicide. Yet here I am, thin, alive and happy. How did I do it? The answer is so simple that it borders on being stupid. **I STUCK TO THE PLAN UNTIL I HAD LOST ALL OF THE EXCESS WEIGHT!**

Weight loss is like getting into an elevator and **STAYING** in it until you get to your floor. If your goal is to reach the fifth floor but you keep getting off on the third floor, whose fault is it that you're not reaching your destination? The answer is obvious. WE are the ones that sabotage our own progress. <u>WE</u> are the ones that give in to the slightest temptation instead of resisting with courage. And you know what? NOBODY can solve this problem for us. There aren't any magic 'gurus' out there who can waive a magic wand and make excess weight disappear. <u>WE</u> are the ones who must grab the bull by the horns and solve the weight problem. I'm going to pour my heart and soul into this material so that you can succeed. But <u>YOU</u> are the one who has to walk through the process. And the sooner you do it, the sooner you can start enjoying your new slim, attractive body. Or you can do nothing and remain fat. There really are no other options. Can you see that? But I have faith that you are here because you have reached the point of no return. I believe in you... and I am certain that, if you follow my plan of action, it won't be long before you begin to see measurable results.

Personal Commitment

I want you to make a commitment with yourself <u>right now</u> that you're going to stop getting off the elevator on the wrong floor. That whatever price needs to be paid to lose the weight and get healthy, that you're willing to pay it. Not later on or down the line, but **NOW**. That was exactly what turned it all around for me. And the catalyst to this turnaround was the daily misery that I was living. Not able to stop eating, I topped 300 pounds and sank into a depression that left me completely paralyzed, defeated and suicidal. It is hard to describe this type of emotional agony. It felt as though my soul was ripped wide open and that all hope for my life was gone.

One particular morning in 1998, I woke up in the living room floor of my apartment covered in urine and vomit. I had eaten three large pizzas the night before and washed them down with a case of beer and a bottle of whiskey. So there I was, a pathetic excuse for a human being... covered in bodily fluids like an animal. That's when the switch inside of me turned. **ENOUGH WAS ENOUGH**. Instead of the usual self-pity, I began to feel righteous anger bubble up inside of me. At that moment I felt like the little boy who is bullied and humiliated at school every day, **UNTIL** one day when he says **NO MORE!** At that moment,

I recall making the commitment with myself to do whatever it took. I was sick of giving in to hunger, to being a slave to my belly and appetites. I didn't care how much hunger and discomfort I had to go through to solve this problem, I was going to do it! I refused to give in... I refused to listen to the mental negativity, to the sadness, anger, boredom, impatience and irritation...

No matter how much my body whined and complained, **I refused to give in to hunger**. I hung on to the diet day after day, week after week, month after month. I closed myself to all other courses of action and put on *'blinders.'* I kept my eyes on the prize - me at 195 pounds instead of 310. And so I hung on and continued to repeat the process daily. Inevitably, 10.5 months later, I reached my goal. And by adopting the same diet and eating structure as a permanent part of my lifestyle, **I have not gained any of the weight back in 12 years**. Was it tough? Yes. Did it hurt? Yes. The discomfort during those first weeks was physical as well as emotional. It was very tough to break free from that destructive lifestyle. Was it worth it? Heck yes!

And here's the kicker: **If you do exactly as I did, you will get exactly what I got!** That's why I called this book **The Permanent Weight Loss Diet**. Because, once you get used to it and make it your own, this diet can stay with you for life. And, if you stick to it, you will <u>never</u> gain back any of the weight that you lose. That has been my experience and I believe it will be yours as well. Simple, straightforward and effective.

Are you ready to cut the crap and do what you have to do? You're a smart person. You know what you have to do. I'm not going to shock you here with any new discoveries. I have a structure and plan, but the rest you already know. You know what it takes to lose weight. Are you finally ready to **DO IT?** If you are, then all you have to do is **follow my lead step-by-step and wait for the miracle to happen**. We're together for the long haul... if it takes three months, if it takes six months, if it takes one year... if it takes two years... stick with me and you **<u>WILL</u>** reach your goal. Let the lazy gluttons continue to bask in their own crap. By purchasing and reading this book, you have made the decision to do this, do it in its entirety... do it without further detours, excuses and **BS** justifications.

Food Addiction

Let me ask you: do you consider yourself to be somebody who just eats too much, or would you say that, maybe, you are addicted to certain foods. The word 'addiction' is ugly, I know. I certainly cannot diagnose you as a food addict. Even if I could I wouldn't do it. That is something that you have to assess yourself in the solitude of your heart and mind. Where do you stand? How bad have your eating habits been? Do you lose control when you eat sometimes?

Do you find it very hard (*almost impossible*) to resist certain foods? Do you find yourself giving in to temptation over and over in spite of your honest desire to stop? If you answered yes to these questions, then it is likely that food addiction is hovering nearby. I came to that conclusion early on. I was a food junkie of the worst kind. **And the US is overrun with food addicts**. This includes those who are morbidly obese, just a little overweight and even thin. **Food is a drug**. It is legal and abundant (*in most* *places*). It is, in essence, the center of human existence. Every occasion, whether joyous or sad, is usually marked with the presence of food and beverage. And, hey... that is great. Food is here for our nourishment and enjoyment. The problem comes when **the instinct to eat exceeds its intended purposes and we become overweight.** If we look at ourselves in the mirror and see rolls of flab, then that is an indication that <u>something has gone wrong</u>.

Somewhere along the line, the urge to eat has taken over and become a compulsion. We have begun to use food irresponsibly. Rather than eating to sustain, nourish and strengthen our bodies, we start using food to medicate emotions, pass the time, deal with boredom, celebrate, mourn... the reasons are endless. I am sure that you can come up with quite a few of your own. **Let me pause real quick and clarify something**: *There are many who suffer from thyroid and other health conditions which can cause weight gain. So I am <u>NOT</u> saying that <u>EVERYONE</u> who is overweight has gotten that way because they are irresponsible, lazy or gluttonous.* However, even in those cases where physical illness causes weight gain, *the person can (usually) still do certain things to help the situation* - be it exercise, dieting, traditional and/or holistic medicine etc. <u>None of us are victims</u>. Some - like me - have to hit a very ugly bottom to finally find the willingness to change. But there is **ALWAYS** something that we <u>**CAN**</u> do.

I have known amazing people who, in spite of being stricken by a terminal illness, remain committed to taking care of their bodies. I've seen men and women with missing limbs ... people who go through life without an arm or a leg. Individuals who are confined to wheelchairs and have very little capacity for independent movement. Nonetheless, they don't allow the handicap to paralyze them. Instead, they continue to take action and do what is within their capacity.

You are **NOT** a victim, a failure, a loser, a weakling or any other trash that the mind may throw your way. You **CAN** do this. And you **ARE** doing it. Otherwise you would not have purchased this book and be taking the time to read it. Now it is time to prepare yourself to go *'all the way.'* Not to lose *'a few* *pounds,'* fall of the wagon, gain them back *(plus a couple more)* and then do it all over again months *(or years)* later, full of guilt and bitterness. No. I want you to be prepared to <u>stay the course without further interruption</u> and lose every last ounce of excess weight. I want this to be the decisive moment in your life. **The time when you get to see yourself in the mirror as you've always dreamed**. <u>Lean and mean</u>. That is what this book is all about.

Discipline and Self-Control

I have found that most of us who have struggled with weight have been very lacking in discipline and self-control. We give in easily, we lack structure and often can live in chaos and disorder. This is not always the case, but many of us have found ourselves completely out of control. So in this book we will work at <u>creating an eating structure</u>. If you really want to lose weight and keep it off, you cannot eat *'whenever.'*

There has to be a meal structure that you follow and adhere to. If we try to do it on our own and refuse structure, we will almost-definitely fail. **So it's not just about**

dieting. It is also about <u>bringing order into our eating habits</u>. It is about learning how to cook our meals and take care of ourselves. It is about letting go of any rebellion and resistance we may have to structure and discipline. I meet many people who come to me desperate because they cannot lose weight. However, the moment I talk about following a structure, they balk and insist on doing things *'their way.'*

Here's the key: You have to be convinced in your heart of hearts that doing it *'your way'* has not worked. You need an eating structure that you can follow and rely on without having to *'guess'* what/when your next meal is going to be. If you can put away resistance and allow yourself to be guided in the way I have described, you will find great peace and freedom. It may take some time for you to get used to having an eating structure and schedule. You may hate it at first. But, as time passes and you begin to see the results, the resistance will fade and you will start to feel better than ever. The obsession with food and eating will subside and you will be free. I have seen this miracle come to pass in the lives of many. Certainly, it came to pass in my own life. And it will in yours as well IF you are willing to set aside the resistance and learn to follow a sound eating structure based on discipline and self-control. Don't worry, I will lay it all out for you in detail. All you have to do is receive the information and take the action. If I did it, so can you!

Chapter 2
Expected Weight Loss

The eating structure that I am going to give you will help you to lose anywhere from 10 to 20 pounds per month (or more). The diet is simple and comprised of common foods that I'm sure you are familiar with. How much weight you lose exactly will depend on your body's reaction. Ten pounds per month is typical, although I have heard of some that have lost 25 and even 30 pounds in one month. **Keep your expectations realistic and move forward with determination**. You **WILL** lose weight. In some cases, the weight loss is slow at first. But it picks up as the weeks go by. Such was the case with me. I lost 14 pounds the first month (*which is still awesome*). The second month I lost 20 pounds, and then the monthly weight loss stabilized at 10-12 pounds. I was very excited because I saw that, with the proper structure, anyone could lose lots of weight fast.

And I have some good news. This is not a typical '*diet*' that starves the living daylights out of you and expects you to do it long-term while whistling and tap dancing. I don't believe in that because it simply isn't realistic. We all have jobs, families and schedules to keep. So we need a diet that produces results, but doesn't cause us to walk around like zombies. I tried that extreme approach many times. And, given, occasionally one may choose to do a fast or some other type of ultra-restrictive short-term calorie restriction. As a matter of fact, I have outlined two of those in **Volume 2 and 3** of this series. Here, however, my aim is to give you a long-term eating structure that will help you to lose weight consistently. And you still get to eat lots of great food and in handsome quantities. I'm not by any means saying that this will be *'easy.'* It will be *'easier'* than perhaps you would expect. But it still will require lots of commitment and willingness to walk through hunger and discomfort. The up side is that your body will get used to it after a few weeks. And, to be sure, the benefits in physical and mental health (*and weight loss*) will totally outweigh the discomfort. So I implore you to follow my instructions to the letter. **Let me be blunt**: The initial phase of any weight loss program is hardest and the one that comes with the most physical and mental discomfort. So, yes... following this diet will initially be challenging. But you've been through that many times before. All that I'm asking is that you put aside excuses and justifications and just stick to the plan. **I implore you to hang on and give yourself wholeheartedly to the task**. Welcome aboard. Let's move forward!

The Great Weight Loss Barrier

The problem, as I said earlier, is that many people begin the weight loss process but quit halfway. They are quickly *'freaked out'* by the discomfort and can't believe *'how hard it is.'* Believe me, I totally understand how disheartening it is to feel that losing weight is out of reach.

Why does this happen? The answer lies with what I call **'The Three Horsemen of The Food Apocalypse -> <u>saturated fats</u>, <u>refined sugar</u> and <u>refined starches</u>. THOSE** are the ones that cause most of the hunger and physical discomfort associated with dieting. Just like a body addicted to nicotine, cocaine or heroin, calorie restriction induces a <u>temporary state of physical and mental crisis</u> that is very tough to navigate. This state is what I call 'The Great Weight Loss Barrier.'

If we can learn to resist the assault from *'the three horsemen'* and ride out the ensuing crisis, we will (*without fail*) cross through the barrier and walk directly into breakthrough territory. It is important to note that, while saturated fats and refined sugar and flour (*as well as caffeine!*) are the primary culprits, too much natural sugar, whole grains and *'healthy'* fats can also cause problems. I have friends who are vegans and vegetarians. Yet they still eat obsessively and are overweight.

You can eat the healthiest and purest foods on the planet. However, if there is no <u>disciplined portion control</u>, the result will (nearly always) be excess weight. Even though crossing this weight loss barrier may sound like a daunting task, I come to you with good news: There <u>IS</u> a solution. And that is **<u>PREPARATION</u>**.

Preparing for Weight Loss

The goal of preparation (*whether you want to lose just a few pounds or have a lot of weight to shed*) is simply this: **Setting Yourself Up to Succeed By Anticipating What Is to Come and – Most Importantly – Being Mentally Ready to Meet The Challenge**

Do you see why this is so important? A warrior who goes into a sword fight with inappropriate weaponry will be injured and defeated because he or she failed to understand the nature of the battle. Starting a weight loss process unprepared and simply *'hoping for the best'* is a recipe for certain failure. Under such circumstances, the person has no defensive weapons or offensive strategy. He or she is entering the arena **blind and without a cane**.

Preparation is needed to gain the upper hand. As I am defining it here, the preparation phase is **the time period that immediately precedes the start of any**

weight loss program. It is the time when you are still carrying the excess weight but have admitted the need for immediate action. This phase of preparation is difficult because goals look very distant - almost unreachable. If you've ever felt that you will never lose weight and have the slim body that you dream of, then you know exactly what I'm talking about.

It is hard to find the motivation to get going because the mind traps us in a delusion that says: "*This weight loss is never going to happen. It is going to take forever to accomplish this. This is an impossible task.*" And little is more discouraging than getting caught in this quicksand of self-hatred and self-pity. We need to start moving, and we need to do it right away. So let's roll up our sleeves and work together on your preparation. :-)

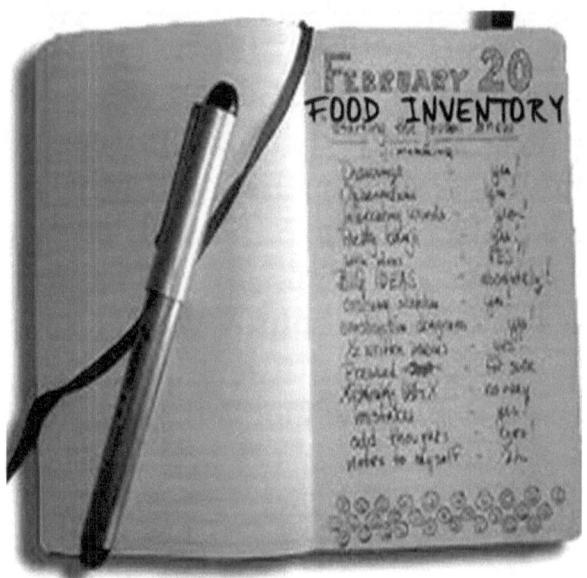

"Putting together a thorough food inventory <u>BEFORE</u> starting any weight loss program greatly increases your ability to go the distance and resist temptation."

Chapter 3
The Food Inventory

The first leg of preparation is **putting together a thorough and honest food inventory**.

<u>**Do This**</u>:

Purchase a journal; a notebook where you can **write about your weight loss process from now on**. Don't get just any cheap, used notebook. I want you to purchase an attractive journal... something that you can identify with. A notebook that appeals to you when you see it. You can find a vast selection online or at most discount stores for very little money, usually around $20.

Sit down in a quiet place where you can remain undisturbed. Turn off your phone and any other distraction (*televisions, music players etc..*)Put pen to paper and start writing an <u>inventory of your eating history</u>. If you've never done this before, it will be very enlightening. It may feel odd initially, perhaps even silly. Ignore the negative thoughts and keep working. People like to talk about food and weight loss. We spend time thinking about food, watching TV shows about eating and looking up the latest restaurant that serves the 'exotic cuisine' that we want to try. Indeed, food takes front and center stage in the human mind.

However, very **few people ever take the time to actually write about their eating habits**. And this 'writing' is extremely helpful when working to achieve both short and long-term weight loss. We need to SEE in black and white the ways in which we have harmed ourselves with food.

When writing, **name the types of foods that you customarily eat. Make sure to also disclose the portions that you consume.** *Think of a common day in your life.* How does it begin? You wake up in the morning, wash up or shower, and then make your way to the kitchen. What did you eat? How much of it did you eat? Would you say that you overate? If so, how did you overeat? *(Example: I had four pieces of toast instead of two, I went overboard on the butter etc..)*

What could you have done better? (*Example: I could have skipped the bacon, watered down the orange juice, had hard-boiled eggs instead of fried, etc..*) Follow this same template with lunch and dinner. List any (*and all*) snacks that you had in between meals. Make sure to take a full inventory of everything that you ate on this particular day. That is one way to do it.

On the other hand, you can mix things up and list the foods that you've eaten in several different days. Think of the worst eating day that you've had in recent memory and take the food inventory. There is no 'wrong' way to do this. **Go with the flow and do it in whichever way comes easiest for you**. What matters is that you get a <u>detailed description</u> of your eating behavior.

You can write: *"In the past year I have abused pastries, particularly birthday cake, muffins, cupcakes and Danish. At times I have eaten an entire cake in one sitting and felt absolutely horrible. My eating is out of control and very harmful,"* and so on. The inventory needs to be thorough. **Leave nothing out**. I want you to <u>see</u> the <u>exact</u>

nature of your eating habits. **Please do not rush**.

You certainly don't have to finish the entire inventory in one session. As a matter of fact, it is better if you do not. Take at least <u>one week</u> to fully catalog your eating behaviors. Be meticulous and explicit in every detail. Once you feel satisfied that the inventory is complete to the best of your ability, ask yourself: For how long has this behavior been going on? Has it been only a few months? Or have I been eating poorly for years... my whole life? The latter was definitely the case with me. When I started to do the inventory, I began to remember being 8 years old and hoarding sweets under my bed so that I could get up when everyone was asleep and gorge.

Internal Reconnaissance

In my personal experience (*and as a weight loss coach*), I have seen time and time again that putting together a thorough food inventory **BEFORE** starting any weight loss program <u>greatly increases</u> the ability to resist temptation, navigate hunger and stay aboard long-term. **Here's why**: The best way to prepare for any meaningful task is to, first of all, have a clear understanding of what it is we're dealing with. That is why, in times of war, soldiers go on reconnaissance missions in enemy territory.

The goal of these missions is to acquire information that can be used to defeat the enemy and, ultimately, win the war. Weight loss is no different. We need fresh and detailed intelligence in writing. To say, "*I am preparing to lose weight,*" is too vague and will not suffice. **I want you to <u>see on paper</u> the <u>precise magnitude</u> of the task at hand**. The food inventory is your <u>ultimate</u> **internal reconnaissance mission**. You are confronting the <u>absolute truth</u> - no matter how ugly and/or hopeless it may seem.

You may have '*known*' all of this in your head. But now, written in the journal and presented before you, it becomes <u>absolute and undeniable</u>. There is no reasoning or justification that can battle against the information you have logged in the food inventory. And, based on the data, the reality is that you **MUST** take action to transcend this foe once and for all. If you don't do whatever it takes to vanquish the destructive eating behavior, it will ride your back for the rest of your days and cripple your life quality. If you fail to overcome, you'll have to deal with the disillusionment of <u>NOT</u> having reached your goals... not having achieved your very best.

Even worse, over time, **you may also have to face adverse and potentially fatal health consequences**. The food inventory represents victory over this enemy. It is top-quality reconnaissance that will help you to win the contest. The challenge in front of you is very clear. And the time has arrived to tackle it head on and, more importantly, triumph over it.

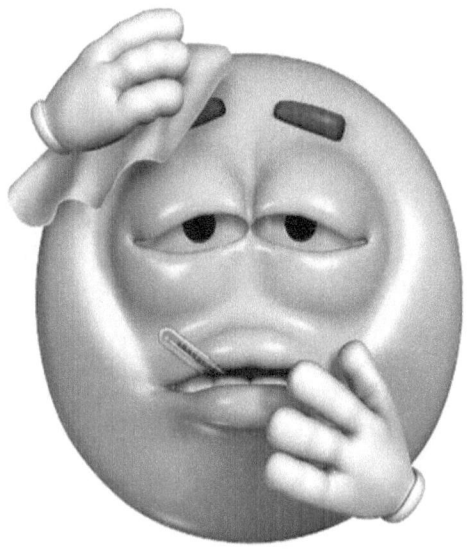

"The body is not used to being deprived of eating whatever it wants and will go through dizzy spells, headache, fever and others symptoms. The best solution is to get as much rest as your schedule allows."

Chapter 4
Weight Loss &
Detox Symptoms

Once you have completed the food inventory to the very best of your ability, you are ready to start step 2 of preparation - understanding the detox/weight loss process. I'm not saying that you *'don't know'* what weight loss is about. What I'm saying is that I want you to become aware of the foes that you will encounter along the way. Let's identify and unmask them now.

When they come, it will be much easier to deal with them. You will discover that you have a great deal more of inner strength than ever before. As I said earlier, the initial stages of weight loss are always the most uncomfortable. I don't have to tell you that. You know what I mean because you've experienced it yourself before.

Earlier we talked about the **'The Three Horsemen of The Food Apocalypse ->** <u>saturated fats</u>, <u>refined sugar</u> and <u>refined starches</u>. All of these foods will be removed from your diet. Consequently, within 48 to

72 hours after you stop their consumption, you will begin to experience what is known as a <u>healing crisis</u>. A healing crisis is a type of *'temporary sickness'* comprised of a variety of symptoms that arise while the body is purging food addictions and excreting toxins through the skin, saliva, urine and feces. In other words, you will be going through withdrawal just like coming off of drugs, nicotine or alcohol.

Didn't food become your drug? Perhaps your addiction to food has been chronic like mine was, or maybe you just eat too much and lack self-control. Whatever the case may be, if you regularly ate any of the *'three horsemen,'* then going through withdrawal is really inevitable. It is important to emphasize that the symptoms experienced are **NOT** an indication that one is getting worse. On the contrary, the presence of a healing crisis indicates that the body is **HEALING**. Hence the name *'healing crisis,'* although it is sometimes also called *'curative crisis.'* The flu-like sickness can last as long as 21 days. However, the worst of the symptoms usually pass within nine days.

These are approximates of course. The initial detox process can be shorter or longer depending on the person's body makeup and overall state of health. Ok, **THESE** are the symptoms and weight loss side-effects that stand between you and your cherished weight loss goals. If you can bear these discomforts and annoyances, then absolutely **nothing will be able to stop you.**

Headaches – This one is especially marked for coffee drinkers, but is also the case for persons who consume large amounts of sugar and alcohol. This symptom can really take a person out of commission. If it gets really bad and you need to take a couple of ibuprofen tablets to ease the pain, then so be it. Two, 200 mg tablets will usually do the trick. Don't take more than four in any given day. Coffee will not be in the list of banned foods. However, caffeine is a stimulant and a drug. Cut down as much as possible. A morning cup of coffee is fine. Three, four, five, six more cups during the day is unacceptable. You will become jittery and be more vulnerable to mood swings and impulsive behavior (more about that shortly). The good news is that headaches rarely last more than 72 hours, if that.

Dizziness – The body is not used to being deprived of eating whatever it wants anytime that it wants. So you may experience some dizzy spells, especially during the first 21 days of detoxification. The best solution for dizziness is to move slowly and get as much rest as your daily schedule allows. Take care to get up very slowly from a sitting position. If you get up too fast, you may feel like you are going to faint. Some have fainted. A little dizziness is to be expected. But severe dizziness is rare because, after all, you will be eating plenty.

Difficulty Performing Basic Tasks – Since you will be eating notably less, it will take some time for the body to adjust, so you will more than likely feel very weak and may have trouble getting around. If you slow down and work at focusing on the individual tasks you are performing, then you will have no problem overcoming this symptom. It is important, however, for you to realize that your body is going through a transition. So you must move slowly and not try to push yourself too hard. You may not be able to function at the same capacity as you are accustomed. Fine. Slow down and give the body time to work.

Weakness means that you need to be extra careful when walking around, and especially when getting up from a sitting position. Avoid harsh and/or abrupt movements. Move slowly, watch your step closely and always have something that you can hang on to if you suddenly feel like you are fainting. This is good advice. One time I totally hit the deck because I got up to quickly from a chair. I missed the corner of the wall by centimeters, but still hit myself quite hard on the floor. This is about improving our health, not about getting hurt. Please be careful. I mean it. Be careful.

Pulsating Hunger Pains that disappear and then re-emerge throughout the day. For some persons, hunger is bad in the morning. But for the vast majority, the **hunger troll shows up <u>mostly at nig</u>**ht. Hunger will always be a part of our lives, and it is our task to master it rather than allow it to enslave us as it **<u>CAN AND WILL</u>** if we let it. In my case, hunger was very strong in the first week to 10 days, and then I found myself getting used to always being 'a little' hungry. After a while, I loved it because I began to feel more alert, more energetic, optimistic...

I slept better. I actually **SLEPT THROUGH THE NIGHT** and woke up feeling terrific. Before the diet, I constantly woke up at night, usually like a raving lunatic wanting to raid the refrigerator. After a while, all of those terrible symptoms diminished and ultimately vanished. I would go to sleep at 11PM, close my eyes and, when I opened them, it was 6AM!

For me, this was nothing less than a total miracle. And I felt great... refreshed and ready to go! All of that just from getting used to eating less and being a little hungry. Much better than getting stuffed like a boar as I used to.

Bad Breath, Metallic Taste in Mouth, White Sticky Film on Tongue – These are all good indications that your body you body is eliminating toxicity. Most of these symptoms pass after nine-to-eleven days.

Bad Breath, I suggest that you get sugarless mints and keep them handy until the process ends.

Metallic Taste In the Mouth usually

means that there are excessive (*and toxic*) heavy metals accumulated in your system. I recall during my first cleansing diet tasting constant sulfur and 'steel' in my mouth for like one week.

White Sticky Film on the Tongue is completely repulsive but necessary. It's just another way for your body to get rid of all of the crap in your body that has kept you addicted to junk and overweight. For these symptoms, the best thing you can do is to keep drinking a lot of water. Make sure to brush your teeth regularly. Keep a travel toothbrush with you if you spend a lot of time out. Mouthwash is also helpful.

Diarrhea or Constipation – All of the fecal matter adhered to your colon will either start gushing out in diarrhea or incite short-term constipation. I know that this is disgusting, but it happens. If you have eaten poorly for a long time, or have simply abused sugar or fat, your body may respond to this cleanse by starting to expel all of the toxic filth in this fashion.

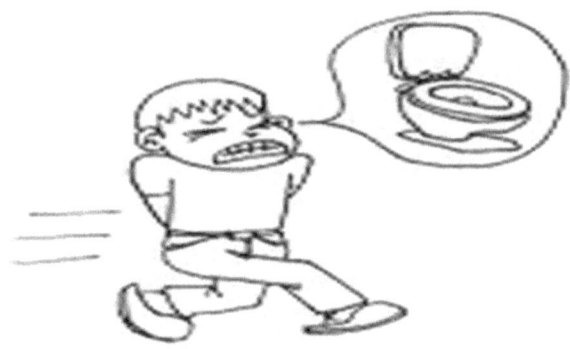

If Diarrhea Strikes, simply continue to follow the cleansing diet as outlined. Should it become severe, see your pharmacist and ask him or her for an over-the-counter recommendation. Continue with the diet. The initial process is a shock to the body, but it will finally get the message and react favorably to what you are doing. If you have diarrhea, make sure to keep yourself hydrated. Make it a point to drink at least one gallon of water daily. Stay close to a bathroom at all times. If you go out, make sure that you are always aware where the nearest restroom is. Seriously, you want to get to the toilet promptly anytime you need to.

If Constipation is The Case: visit your local pharmacy and ask your pharmacist about a stool softener. I personally use a herbal laxative called **Herbs & Prunes**. It works like a charm every time and is not harsh on my stomach. Take one tablet to start. Do not exceed four tablets in one day. But do this only if you fail to eliminate anything for at least three days. Give your body enough time to do it on its own.

Irritability / Mood Swings – If you have ever seen The Flintstones, you may remember Fred walking around growling on the episode where he is placed on a diet. Sooooo, be prepared to be a little *"short-fused"* during this time of heavy-duty preparation. Be aware that you will not be as patient as you normally would be. Tell your loved ones not to take it personally if - initially - you are less social that what they are accustomed. This Is Normal & Will Pass! Mood swings also can include boredom, impatience and frustration with the weight loss process.

Facial Puffiness & Feeling Bloated – This symptom is much more marked for persons who consume large amounts of salt and/or sugar. The body is, in essence, disoriented when sugar and salt intake is so minimized and many times retains water for some days and becomes "*hyper-sensitive*" and toxic. I personally was bloated to the max like the Stay Puft Marshmallow man. So being puffy was nothing new. It looked like somebody had stuck huge balloons on my cheeks. It was hideous. The diet took care of that and my face today is that of a normal human being rather than a cartoon character.

That's pretty much it. Now tell me: **which of the symptoms mentioned in this section is greater than you?** Which of these will you permit to knock you off course? The truth is that **NONE** of these symptoms is bigger or stronger than you. You have what it takes to resist, endure and walk through <u>all</u> of them. And you can accomplish this, <u>WITHOUT</u> having to quit or fall off the wagon. Are you going to '*die*' if you don't eat the junk that the body is asking for? You do not need to '*medicate*' any of your emotions with food. There is nothing to '*fix.*' All you have to do is be still, continue to move forward and wait for the storm to pass. Indeed, you are out of excuses. I have listed here pretty much every challenge that you will experience during the entire weight loss process. And, as far as I can see, the only one that can stand in your way now is you. Go through this section and read each of the symptoms several times. I am sure that you recognize most, if not all Staying the course **IN SPITE OF** these challenges is the key to success. You have the information. You know what you have to do. The only real choice that you have at this point is to <u>push through and overcome</u>. Alright, let's begin!

Chapter 5
The Grocery List

Now it's time to go shopping, to begin the amazing journey of transforming your eating habits. First I am going to give you the shopping list. Then we can look at the menu in detail, and - after that - I will give you tips on how to prepare the meals as quickly and easily as possible. As I said at the start of the book, the best way to lose weight and keep it off is to have an eating structure. And yes... that means that you will be cooking for yourself. Even if you have a loved one who is willing to cook for you, I strongly encourage you to start by doing it yourself. The food preparation process, over the course of weeks, will impact you very positively. You will begin to see that you **CAN** maintain a clean diet. Cooking my own meals is something that gave me a great deal of self-esteem and satisfaction. What was even more amazing was when the pounds started to drop off. Having abused food for so long, it was hard to believe that I actually was not only cooking, but cooking meals that were good for me!. That was a <u>HUGE</u> departure from being locked in my apartment for weeks, without bathing or shaving and constantly ordering pizzas and Chinese food. This was different. This was **me doing good things for me**. Perhaps for you cooking isn't a big deal. That's great. You're way ahead of the game. But most overweight people that I talk to tell me that they only know how to cook junk. One lady actually broke down in tears when she first started to cook for herself. "I can't believe I'm actually taking care of myself... being responsible for my health," she said. "What about you? Are you ready to start taking care of yourself? Yes, I believe that you are. In the past I was a slave to whatever other people were cooking. Or I was a slave to my own apathy and laziness, which would lead me to eat the worst foods possible, "because I hate cooking." But let me assure you. When I talk about cooking, I don't mean that you will be expected to prepare complicated meals. The diet is very simple. Basic cooking is all that will be required. Ok, enough yapping. Let's check out the shopping list.

Shopping List

* **Boneless Chicken Breast** - Try to find a bag with six or ten breasts, I often go to the

freezers and grab a large back of breasts from there. You need to have your protein, so stock up on the chicken.

* Extra Lean Ground Turkey Breast (*no deli turkey*) Ground turkey has been my saving grace, let me tell you. I was so confused and whacked out of my mind when I first started doing this, that even cooking a piece of chicken on the skillet was difficult. Ground turkey is very easy to cook, can be mixed into eggs for breakfast... and it basically is my lifeline. When buying ground turkey, but the one with the least amount of fat please. Don't just grab the first serving you come across. Stop and read the labels... find out how much fat it contains. I would say that a package of ground turkey that is 85% meat, 15% fat should be fine. You can drain the excess fat later. The 'fat-free' ground turkey can get quite expensive and, to be honest, it tastes like the sole of a shoe. It is very tough, dry and not very tasty at all. Stick to the 85/15 for now.

* Egg Whites; Yes, real eggs are out. We want the protein from the egg whites, but not the fat and cholesterol from the yolk. I had a real hard time letting go of eggs because I ate them almost daily since I was a toddler. I loved eggs, but I had some form of asthma or allergic condition, so I was not allowed to eat eggs. I would still eat them, however. Even if I had to get up while everyone was sleeping, I **WOULD** eat eggs! As you can see, my tendency toward rebellion, wanting to do things 'my way," and disregarding council were alive and well inside of me. So no eggs please. Egg whites are fine. I have gotten used to them and no longer obsess over real eggs like I used to **Note**: I use the liquid egg whites that come in a box because all I have to do is pour into the pan and cook. Besides, I always make a huge mess separating the yolk! :-)

* Low Sodium Tuna Fish

Note: This kind usually can be found in envelopes rather than cans. You're going to be getting your sodium directly from the foods that you will eat. No salt is to be added to any food at any time for any reason. That's not cause for you to give up and throw in the towel, is it? Right now, we are barely getting started. We need to lay a strong foundation, and that includes foods that you must avoid. But that is no surprise to you. You know what you have to do. I'm here as your guide and facilitator... as your coach. But you and you alone are the one that needs to keep walking forward. l

* **Fresh Fish** (*Tilapia and Grouper. Salmon Once Weekly ONLY*) - Fish can be expensive, so what I do is I buy it frozen from the supermarket refrigerators. Most markets have a decent variety of frozen fish. Tilapia is great and very lean. Grouper would also do the trick. You don't have to fill an entire cart with fish, but by all means pick up a few bags. Of course if you can afford to buy wild, fresh fish... then that is definitely the way to go. Farm fish give me the creeps, to be honest. Those fish are given all kinds of pesticides. Many are even given artificial colors. Yes, if the fish is orange... the orange was man-made. The fish itself did not acquire that color on its own.

* **Baked Potatoes** -are my saviors. I just love them. I can come in from the street famished and all I have to do is nuke one of those puppies for ten minutes and it's good to go.

* **Sweet Potatoes** - I love sweet potatoes as

well. Very easy to prepare. Potatoes and sweet potatoes are good starches... complex carbohydrates that will give you clean energy. There are potatoes that come wrapped up in plastic ready to be tossed into the microwave. While that IS very handy, these supermarkets want like $2 for each. Just on principle, I won't pay it. Maybe where you live these pre-wrapped potatoes are cheaper.

Quaker Oats (100% Whole Grain, Quick Oats). Another complex carb that I rely on every day - especially in the mornings. Get a good amount.

Cream of Wheat (White Box) Get a good amount as well so that you can mix these up in your breakfasts.

Cream of Rice - all great stuff, awesome complex carbs rich in fiber... clean food that will cleanse and transform your body.

Pasta (Only Whole Grain or Whole Wheat - No Egg Noodles) I'm a pasta freak. So the rule of thumb is to stick ONLY to whole grain or whole wheat. Anything that is enriched (white pasta) should be deemed garbage and not consumed.

***Brown Rice** - I love my brown rice, especially the boil-in-the -bag type which requires no cooking. I am terrible cooking rice, that's the truth. It nearly always comes out mangled and chewy... a total freak show. So I stick with the boil-in-the-bag, and it works very well.

***Fresh Green Vegetables** (*Broccoli, Carrots, Cauliflower* etc...) **Note**: These are great for steaming. I usually purchase the bags that come with them already pre-mixed. You will find a lot of different veggie combinations to choose from in these pre-mixed bag selections. I like these because all I have to do is wash them and steam them. Again... keeping it simple, right?

***Balsamic Vinegar and Olive Oil:** These two are going to be your salad dressing from now on. All other dressings are banned. Most of them are packed with sugar and fat. Do NOT add any dressing other than the olive oil and balsamic vinegar. I was a Blue Cheese nut. I'd eat it every day... I'd put Blue Cheese on my cereal if you let me. Well, not really... but you get the idea. When I was first confronted with having to stop using it,

I kicked and screamed. I admit it. I talked about lazy gluttons at the start of the book. Well, it takes one to know one. I had a hard time using only olive oil and balsamic vinegar. However, today I wouldn't trade them for anything in the world. I look at a bottle of blue cheese now and it sickens me that I was eating all of that fat and sugar.

* **Garlic and Onion Powder** -Ok, these are the puppies here that you will use to spice the food. But you have to make sure that you get the garlic and onion powder, NOT the garlic or onion salt. In addition, pick up a few bottles of **Mrs. Dash No Salt All-Purpose Seasoning.** Those three are basically the only seasonings that I have used in many years. I no longer add salt to anything. There are different kinds of Mrs. Dash. Pick the one you like the most. I like the Garlic & Herbs mixed with the garlic and onion powder. They come together very well and do the job. I don't miss salt at all. Give it time and you'll get to the same point, trust me.

*Enricos No Salt-No Fat Spaghetti Sauce** (*Or Any Other No-Salt Brand You Find*) Alright, this Enrico's sauce is very good.

However, it is often a pain in the neck to find. Go to the pasta aisle in your local supermarket. If you don't see it there, see if they have a 'specialty pasta' display anywhere in that vicinity. If not, they may have it in another aisle under 'heath foods.' Ask a supermarket clerk for assistance. Tell him or her that you need a pasta sauce that comes with NO SALT ADDED. If they don't have Enrico's, he or she may direct you to another brand. Just make sure that the pasta sauce has no salt added.

Stevia Sweetener (*No Equal or Splenda*) I realize that you may want to have a cup of coffee or tea in the morning, or that you may want to sweeten up the oatmeal. I mean, who wants to eat oatmeal plain, right? Might as well eat a piece of cardboard. Yes, we're going to go with the Stevia sweetener, By NO MEANS do I ever want you to consume Equal or Splenda. I'm not going to get into that speech right now. Suffice it to say that I don't want you to put any toxins in your body. And those artificial sweeteners are toxic and harmful. Stevia is alright... it is a leaf. It does tend to have a slight bitter under taste. So at first you may be cursing me from afar when you use it.

But in a few weeks you'll totally get used to it.

*Any Sugar-Free and Low-Sodium Salad Dressing - Going back to dressings real quick, I had forgotten that there ARE some brands out there that come with no salt or sugar added. If you take some time and peruse the displays, I'm sure you will find something that will work. Ask the supermarket clerk for help. It took me about an hour to find my Olde Cape Cod Raspberry Light dressing. Look for that same on where you live and see if you can live with it. It is the one with the lowest amount of salt and sugar that I found

*Fresh Strawberries or Cantaloupe - Good stuff. We are cutting out refined sugar, but natural sugar from fruits (in moderation) will be just fine. Strawberries and cantaloupe are two of the fruits with the least amount of sugar.

*Hunts No Salt Ketchup (*If you like ketchup*) Maybe you don't eat ketchup. I, on the other hand, have been on ketchup since I was a toddler. But I only use it occasionally, and I stick to the no salt kind.

*Gilda Toasted Bread (*no salt or sugar added*). These toasts are great to kill the hunger in between meals when used sparingly. They can usually be found in the bread or health-food aisle of most supermarkets. I can't tell you how many times a Gilda toast has saved me from disaster. We need to be ready because we know that the body will be complaining a lot, and the mind will be trying to harass you - talk you into giving up. We know that it is going to happen. The difference is that we are preparing. We will be ready. **YOU** will be ready.

*Seltzer Water (Sparkling Water/Club Soda) - If you have visited my website FitnessThroughFasting.com and read some of the content, you may have heard me mention seltzer water. Years ago, while I was in the middle of some very tough hunger pangs and detox symptoms, a friend of mine just casually said "Here, drink this." The moment the effervescence hit my stomach, it was like magic. The hunger calmed down almost right away and the symptoms became much more tolerable. I'm telling you, seltzer is the bomb. It is a crucial weapon to have in our arsenal, so make sure to stock up with a 24-pack at least.

*Decaffeinated Green Tea - Green tea is yet another weapon that we want to have in our arsenal. Green tea has body-heating properties which help to give you a pep of energy as well as accelerate weight loss. I am not putting all of my bank on the 'weight loss' aspect of the tea. It is true that it has body-heating properties. And when we are dieting, hungry and weak, we need an ally such as this to come and restore us.

*Decaffeinated Coffee - I mention 'decaf' here because, in my process, I decided that I wanted to be free of all stimulants, including caffeine. I always ended up drinking more than I should, I'd get all jittery and end up succumbing to a food temptation mostly because of frustration and irritability. I would prefer if you joined me and let go of all stimulants as well. It may seem like an impossible request at first, but today... I don't miss coffee one bit. And I was a massive coffee drinker. Obviously I cannot force you to stop drinking coffee if that is what you wish to do. But I CAN tell you that as long as you have stimulants in your body, the risk will always be present that something could set you off and lead you to do something foolish.

Chamomile Tea (*To Help soothe nighttime hunger and help in case of insomnia*) This tea is absolutely magnificent. I rely on it to help settle me down at night. I'm a nighttime person, so many times I have a hard time turning in at a decent hour. As we talked about earlier, when we are dieting, a lot of toxins are released into the bloodstream while the body detoxifies. Sometimes, this release of toxins can cause insomnia, a sense of mania or, as it happened to me, nightmares. Chamomile helps to pretty much neutralize all of that unpleasantness so that I can lay down and get some rest.

* **Valerian Root** (*To Help You Sleep*) Here's another excellent herbal supplement. This sucker works. It knocks me out every time. Take one or two tablets if you are having trouble sleeping.

Tryptophan (*This is an amino acid that also acts as a mood stabilizer and could help* *you sleep at night if you find yourself restless*) But a bottle of the 500 mg tablets. Tryptophan has a very calming effect. Sometimes when dieting, we may get really frazzled about a situation, or we may simply fall into a very foul mood. We may wish to lash out at "the other people who can eat and I have to stick to this BS structure." When I get into those dark spaces, taking one tablet of Tryptophan can help to calm me and give me the window I need to escape from the onslaught.

A Lot of Food!

That's it! When I first give this list to personal coaching clients, they ask me if somehow I made a mistake and gave them too much food. Yes, this is a good amount of food, right? Even today, I am amazed when I walk to the kitchen table with this plate packed with meat, pasta, salad and veggies. This is good eating. This is what the body deserves. And even with all of this food, you are going to start losing a lot of weight.

The whole point is **NOT** to **NOT** eat, but rather to **EAT SMART**. I want you to be as comfortable as possible and, even more, I want you to be able to get through your daily schedule without dragging your elbows on the ground. You still are going to feel the pinch, don't get me wrong. This is a very solid fat-burning diet, so you will have moments when hunger and other symptoms come around to holler at you. But whatever you go through will be tolerable because you are preparing yourself to the ultimate level. Let's finalize the shopping list by making sure that we are **CRYSTAL CLEAR** on foods that are banned, as well as foods that should be limited...

Banned Foods List:

*****Salt** - you get plenty of it from the foods that you will eat. When I first started my diet years ago, I was kind of shocked to see that salt was banned. I spoke against it actually. I have come to realize that the foods we eat all have sodium, and that a healthy adult really has no need for 'salt' except to make the food taste better. In addition, when I stopped using salt, I immediately dropped like 15 pounds. It was mostly water weight, but it showed me that I was retaining a LOT of liquids, and that was greatly due to my abuse of salt and seasonings.

***Sugar** - absolute trash, toxic to the body... good for nothing - stay away! I could write pages and pages about sugar. I am sure that you yourself can admit that this is one of our greatest (if not our greatest) enemy. I mean it. Enemy. Any prolonged return to sugar will, sooner or later, result in a full-blown relapse and the regaining of the weight that I've lost, I don't kid myself by thinking that "I'm cured." I still am susceptible to sugar and to binging. What keeps me free is not to put sugar into my body... period. I can't draw the same conclusion for you, but I am certain that you probably have your own stories to tell about sugar and how it has affected your weight, life and health.

***Fried Foods** - Absolute filthy grease fest that leads to obesity and other diseases.

***Cheese** - Cheese is great but it has way too much fat. For the time being, steer clear. Later on, once you reach your weight loss goal, you will be able to have treats from time to time. So don't let the mind start telling you that your 'life is over' because you can't eat this or that. Just tell the mind to shut up and keep moving forward. Works like a charm for me.

***Dairy Products** - dairy has a lot of fat, is high in sugar content and has been known to cause digestive system inflammation. But I'm not totally heartless. Stock to non-fat milk, how's that? Anything above non-fat is banned.

***Red Meat** - I personally don't have anything against red meat. In fact, I have been known to eat a piece of meat on rare occasion. Right now, we are banning it because it has a lot of fat, and because I want your digestive system to be given easy food to digest. Later on you can have a piece of meat here and there if you want. Right now... it's banned.

***Alcohol** - Alcohol is packed with empty calories. Calories with **ZERO** nutritional value. And booze turns to sugar. Bad all over. If you drink frequently, cut it down to a minimum. You're doing this for your health and to reach a goal that is important to **YOU**.

If you have to go a few months without drinking, your arm is not going to fall off. You'll live. A cup of wine with dinner is fine, but nothing more than that at this juncture.

* **Butter or Margarine** - As they say in New York, "Forget about it!!!" Butter and margarine are pure fat and we don't want it.

*__Fruit Juices__ - If you read the label of most orange juice brands, you will see that the sugar content is through the roof. Yes, it is natural sugar, but sugar nonetheless. You can have one glass of juice in the morning, but you need to water it down 50/50. Drinking straight juice at this phase is basically like injecting blubber directly into your belly. Stay away. Drink veggie juice instead...but make sure that it is the low sodium veggie juice. :-)

*__White Enriched Bread__ - That stuff is like dropping a ball of cement into the stomach. That white flour, doughy garbage really is terrible for human health. I was going to ban all breads, but I remembered that the Ezekiel brand (green bag) is actually very good. You can eat one slice here and there as partial replacement to your carbohydrate servings. We'll get into all of that in just a minute.

*Junk Food of ANY Kind.** I think that it definitely goes without saying that junk food is out. And not just out for a little while. Hopefully, it is out of your life for good. That crap is like wearing a ball and chain. It enslaves us to cravings that are never satisfied and only get stronger and more violent.

Foods to Limit

*Fruits (Stick To Strawberries or Cantaloupe)**
* Tomatoes
* Peas or Corn
* Olive Oil

Chapter 6
Take Immediate Action

So there you go. Take this list with you to the supermarket and fill it as soon as you can. **Today would be best**. You already have cut out the junk that you identified in your food inventory. We have to move quickly and give you the proper eating structure so that you can get into your *'pace'* and start seeing results.

o go fill the shopping list and come back when you're done so we can look at how you will implement the daily meal plan. **I suggest that you take a friend with you to the supermarket to give you support.** You already have cut out the junk from your diet and may be feeling hunger inching its way to the top. You don't want this trip to the store to turn into a binging debacle. So **protect yourself and take someone with you to keep you in check and give you support.**

One More Item: We are going to work on portion control. Therefore, you will need a kitchen scale to weigh some of the foods that you're going to eat. I suggest that you get a digital scale with large numbers for easy viewing.

Get one that weighs in ounces since that is the measuring system that I will be using in the meal structure below. I have owned the **My Weigh KD-7000** digital scale for several years and I love it. It runs around $40 and reads in grams, ounces, pounds and kilograms. But, if you don't already have a scale, please make sure to get one.

Chapter 7
Diet Implementation

Ok, you have purchased all of the groceries needed for the diet as well as the scale, right. Now we have are ready to get into the implementation. How are you feeling? I want to make this process as easy as possible for you. Therefore, rather than putting together a menu based on what I normally eat, I have actually done something better. I've put together a chart for males, and another one for females. Simply follow the directions on the corresponding one and you're on your way.

This structure is effective because **<u>YOU</u>** can pick yourself what you want to eat (*based on the food groups and allowed portions*). This makes it **<u>MUCH</u>** easier because all you have to do is stick to the correct quantities of each food group ... period. In my opinion, **diets that try to make one eat this or that usually don't work because we are individuals and each have our own tastes and preferences.** So this diet aims to give you as much flexibility as possible to eat what you like, and eat **A LOT**!. The most important part of this process is to stick to the allowed foods and quantities. Alright? Let's check it out and get going. :-)

Note: The meal structures below are based on a '*daytime*' schedule. However, I realize that many people may have a schedule that starts in the afternoon or even at night. That is fine. **Follow the meal times based on your actual schedule**. For example, if you work swing shift and don't get up until around 11:00AM, you can have your breakfast meal at noon, and move forward from there. What I'm saying is this: make this cleansing diet **YOURS**. Use it based on **YOUR** schedule and the realities of your daily life. It will work just fine. The most important part is to stick to the food types and quantities and **NEVER** touch anything that is on the list of banned foods.

Serving Sizes

Protein

Egg Whites	**4-5**
Turkey Breast	**4 oz.**
(NOT Cold Cuts)	
Chicken Breast	**4 oz.**
Fish	**5-6 oz.**
(Limit Salmon & Shellfish)	
Tuna Fish	**4-5 oz.**
(Low Sodium)	

Carbohydrates

Baked Potato	**3-4 oz.**
Oatmeal	**1/2 cup.**
(Dry Weight)	
Sweet Potato	**5-6 oz.**
Cream of Wheat	**1-2 oz.**
Cream of Rice ...	**1-2 oz.**
Pasta	**-1.5 oz.**
(Dry Weight)	
Brown Rice	**1/2–3/4 cups**
(Cooked)	
Gilda Toast	**Two Slices**

Meal Plan: Male

Reduce Body Fat & Cleanse

Breakfast: Start -> 8AM
2 Servings of Protein
1-2 Servings of Carbohydrates

Lunch: 4 Hours -> Noon
2 Servings of Protein
1-2 Servings of Carbohydrates

Afternoon: 4 Hours -> 4PM
2 Servings of Protein
1 Serving of Carbohydrates

Dinner: Finish -> 8PM
2 Servings of Protein
NO Carbohydrates

Eat NOTHING else until breakfast the next day. This gives the body 12 hours daily of fasting to digest, detox and heal.

Meal Plan: Female

Reduce Body Fat & Cleanse

Breakfast: Start -> 8AM
1 Servings of Protein
1-2 Servings of Carbohydrates

Lunch: 4 Hours -> Noon
1 Servings of Protein
1-2 Servings of Carbohydrates

Afternoon: 4 Hours -> 4PM
1 Servings of Protein
1 Serving of Carbohydrates

Dinner: Finish -> 8PM
1 Servings of Protein
NO Carbohydrates

Eat NOTHING else until breakfast the next day. This gives the body 12 hours daily of fasting to digest, detox and heal.

Chapter 8
Additional Instructions

All measurements equal one serving.

Pasta: Use No Salt Spaghetti Sauce or No Salt Salsa. Steer clear of parmesan cheese, salt or any other seasoning apart from the ones in the shopping list (Mrs. Dash, garlic powder, onion powder etc...)

Vegetables & Salad: Fresh green vegetables and green salads can be eaten at any and in all meals. <u>NO</u> canned vegetables. <u>NO</u> bottled salad dressings aside from the low-sodium low-sugar ones in the shopping list. You can also use balsamic vinegar and/or fresh lemon juice.

Beverages: You may drink water, unsweetened tea, decaffeinated coffee (you can use the 'half-caffeine' type to ease detox symptoms) and seltzer water (sparkling water, club soda). Moreover, you are allowed one eight-ounce glass of non-fat milk daily. You can have the milk in your oatmeal, coffee or as a stand-alone glass at night before going to bed.

Green Tea Afternoons

The toughest stretch of time to get through while on the cleansing diet is usually afternoons. At around 2pm, you may find yourself feeling very hungry, weak, grouchy and just not at all with the program.

When this happens, we need to pull out a very special weapon, and that is **decaffeinated green tea**.

Drinking pure oolong tea or green tea extract - *a more concentrated form of oolong tea* - will give you energy and calm physical discomfort. The green tea leaf has large quantities of phytochemical polyphenols called flavonols, commonly known as catchetins.

According to a recent green tea study by the Linus Pauling Institute at Oregon State University, green tea fosters weight loss because **the body starts using greater amounts of energy after it is consumed.**

This is a direct result of the catchetins' intrinsic fat oxidation and body heating properties.

In short, green tea can help a lot. You can find a good selection at most supermarkets.

Have some baggies on you wherever you go so that you can offset that annoying afternoon sinking spell. But please make sure to only get decaf green tea if at all possible.

The Seltzer Weapon

You should be **constantly drinking water throughout the day**. Any time hunger comes around, fill up an eight-ounce glass of water and <u>drink it down</u>.

Have another one for good measure. Every night by 8 or 9pm, you should have consumed as close to a full gallon of water as possible.

Yes, you will be urinating **<u>A LOT</u>**, but your kidneys will receive one heck of a detox cleanse.

In addition to water, I recommend seltzer water (*sparkling water, club soda*) with a squeeze of lemon or lime. **Seltzer will help**

to calm hunger pangs and settle the stomach.

Wherever you go, take a small cooler with you packed with ice, drinking water and a few bottles of seltzer.

You want to be prepared at all times to deal with any symptoms or hunger that may emerge.

Don't overdo it with the seltzer, but drink as many as four bottles daily - especially during the first days when hunger and discomfort are at their peak.

And do not drink sodas *(cola)* of any kind, even if it is diet.

In Case of Insomnia

In the first days of the cleansing diet, it is possible that you may have a hard time falling asleep. The reason for this is that the body is releasing large amounts of toxins into the bloodstream and your entire body is on overdrive, working to heal, cleanse and burn fat.

Not being able to sleep can be very annoying, particularly if you have to wake up early in the morning to go to work or fulfill some other obligation. Therefore, if you find yourself tossing and turning, **get up and make yourself a cup of chamomile tea with a squeeze of lemon or lime.** Sorry, no honey or sugar.

Chamomile tea is very soothing and will help you go to sleep. In addition, you can have **one 500 mg tablet of the amino acid Tryptophan**. I use Tryptophan all of the time. Together with chamomile tea, it works like a charm and does not leave residual drowsiness when you wake up in the morning. As an alternative to Tryptophan, you can take a tablet of Valerian Root about half an hour before retiring. In the event that you find yourself still unable to fall asleep, **the best suggestion I can give you is to have a book handy that you can read or, even, go for a short walk around the block.** I took many, many walks during the initial phase of cleansing and found that it helped ease the cravings and relax me so I could fall asleep.

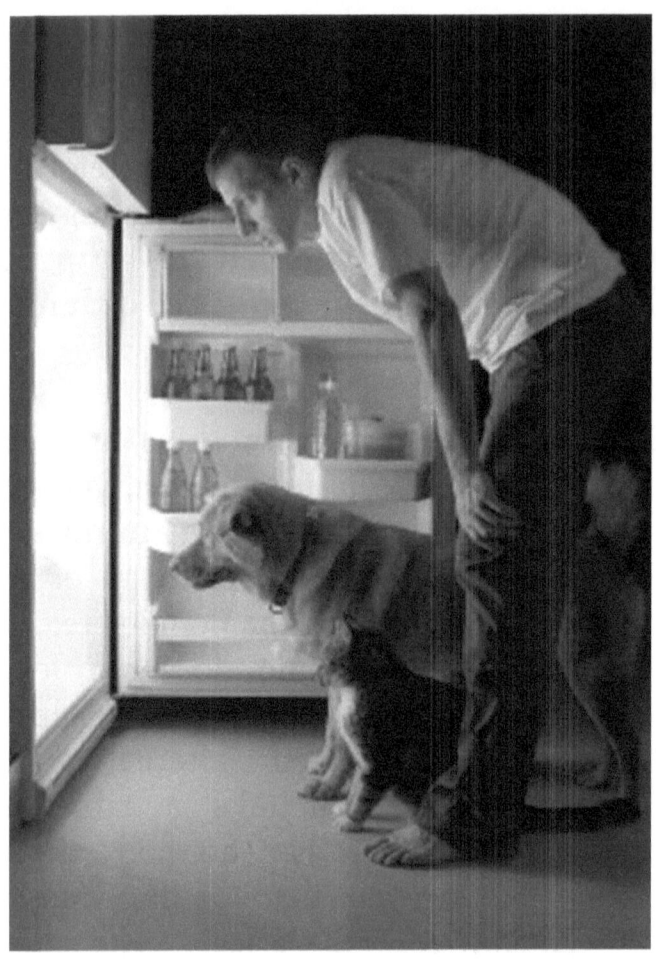

"For some, the biggest challenge is waking up in the middle of the night with monstrous, nearly blinding cravings."."

Night Cravings

For some, the biggest challenge is waking up in the middle of the night with monstrous cravings. At this hour, part of the mind is asleep. Hunger may want to take advantage of that and lead you to eat. So you must be cautious and ever vigilant. If you find yourself in this situation, drink a large glass of water and/or have some seltzer with lime. **I like to keep a gallon of water next to my bed so I can grab it immediately.**

Key Tip: **DO NOT** walk to the kitchen!! The kitchen if **OFF LIMITS!!!** Go to the bathroom, living room or study, but the focus during these night attacks is to <u>NOT</u> go to the kitchen for any reason whatsoever! Have water and/or seltzer close to you – preferably next to your bed on the night table. Yes, the water will probably be warm. <u>DO NOT</u> walk to the kitchen to get ice either! **That is a trick of the mind to get you to open the refrigerator where you will be vulnerable.**

So drink one or two large glasses of water and go back to bed. Repeat this as often as necessary. The wave of cravings may initially come two, three or even four times or more. OR, you may not get hit with cravings but, instead, find yourself constantly getting up to urinate. In either case, the result may be that, during those first days, you do not get a great deal of sleep. Hang in there and stick to the instructions. All of this will soon pass and you will start to feel better and better.

In The Morning

Morning is (usually) the most comfortable part of the day. You probably won't feel hunger or any other symptom for several hours. Nothing matches the awesome feeling of waking up, felling light and knowing that you didn't give in to temptation the previous night.

Your first task upon arising (before breakfast), is to drink **TWO** large glasses of water. You will feel the water going down the belly. It is a great feeling. Drinking water in the morning induces excellent bowel movements which help to expedite the detox process.

Additional Tips: To move your bowels even more, you can squeeze lemon juice into a cup of warm water and add a touch of raw honey with a pinch of rock salt. You can drink one or two cups as soon as you get up. Or, if you feel daring, you can drink the two cups as a full replacement of your breakfast meal. Another alternative is to mix organic lemon juice, warm water, a little maple syrup and a pinch of cayenne pepper. This is similar to the mixture that is used as part of the Master Cleanse diet, a popular fasting detox regimen.

If you are having regular and thorough bowel movements on your own, then there really is no need to drink any of these additional concoctions. I give them to you as an FTY and so that you can be aware of the various choices that you have if you start struggling with constipation.

Chapter 9
Food Preparation

Now let me share with you some tips on food preparation and the diet in general. You can make the dinner salad as large as you want it. The rest of the meals are to be followed <u>exactly</u> as written. Drink only water with the meals. Normally, an advanced cleansing diet would cut out even the meat. However, for the purposes of initial preparation this combination works very well.

If You're a Vegetarian

If you're a vegetarian, you can replace the poultry and fish with **plant-sourced protein in small quantities**. The best choices are well-cooked whole grain and bean combinations. The smaller the bean, the easier it is to digest.

Mung beans are well-known for their cleansing and protective attributes. Whole mung beans can be sprouted and eaten like a vegetable. Brown rice and red lentils are another good protein combination. My personal favorite is tofu. Nuts and seeds also provide protein but are high in fat and best eaten fresh in very small quantities (1/4 cup). With these variations, you will have no trouble completing the cleansing diet as a vegetarian.

Seasoning Fish & Poultry

Seasoning the Fish and/or Chicken: Make sure the fish or chicken pieces have been thoroughly washed. Squeeze fresh lemon on both sides of the meat.

Then you can add the customary garlic and onion powder and/or Mrs. Dash salt-free seasoning. When at the supermarket, spend some time in the seasoning products aisle and pick out your choice of the salt-free alternatives. A final option is to add a very light touch of apple cider vinegar for additional taste.

'Ziplocking' Portions

To expedite the food preparation process, I recommend that you pre-season enough meat (fish, chicken and ground turkey) for 7 days' worth of meals. Put the 6 or 8 oz portions in small zip lock bags. I keep enough meat in the fridge to last me around three days and freeze the rest.

I love *ziplocking (not a real word, I made it up)* because it gives the meat time to fully marinate. Also, it frees up my time because I don't have to go through the cutting, weighing and seasoning process every single day. Cutting, weighing, seasoning and bagging enough meat for seven days usually takes me around 25 minutes. Once it's done... You're good for an entire week.

To eat, all you have to do is pull out one of the baggies from the fridge and toss the meat on the pan to cook. I put labels on the zip lock bags and write in the exact weight (*digital kitchen scales are awesome*) as well as the date in which the meat was bagged. Dating the meat is practical because you want to make sure that older bags are always used first.

Every morning after breakfast, I take a few baggies from the freezer and move them to the fridge to cover my meals for another day or two. Simple tips, but they make the meal preparation process A LOT easier.

Cooking The Meat

To Cook The Meat: Spray a light coat of canola Spam spray on a cooking pan. Spam is the only kind of oil that you will be using during this cleansing diet. Turn the stove to medium heat. Place the meat on the pan. Allow it to brown on both sides with the pan partially covered.

A 6-to-8-ounce piece of lean fish or poultry should not take more than 15 minutes to fully cook on both sides. You want to make sure the meat is cooked thoroughly so as to ensure that all bacteria are destroyed.

About Caffeine

If you are an avid coffee drinker as I was, then eliminating this beverage from your diet completely will be a challenge during the next two to four days. You will experience marked headaches and probably be in an overall cranky mood. **Caffeine is a drug**.

I suggest that, if the headaches become unbearable, make a <u>small amount</u> of very watered down coffee and drink it to soothe. Do it first thing in the morning if that is when you usually drink the most coffee. **My headaches were massive and this helped a lot**. During the day, what worked for me best was to carry some aspirin or other pain reliever and take a few tablets when the pain struck. See your pharmacist and ask for a recommendation that is best for you. Withdrawal from caffeine is a very important part of this detox process, so I encourage you to do it!

I am not telling you to give up coffee for good. That is up to you, although I do believe you would be better off to do so, or at least keep its consumption to a bare minimum. I was a coffee fanatic. Yet, once I got used to drinking non-caffeinated tea, I felt better than ever and did not miss coffee at all. The good news is that withdrawal from caffeine does not usually last longer than three days and the headaches will soon go away.

Be Good to Yourself

If you stumbled and were not able to complete the cleansing, please don't worry.

Yes, I know – it is a tough call. But it is not impossible. So... just because you fell short of the goal and were unable to complete it on one particular try, you should not feel that you failed. **This distinction is crucial because it is at this point that many people give up**. They feel that losing weight is too hard or impossible. That is simply **NOT TRUE**!

You are continuing to learn and position yourself for breakthrough. This process is challenging but highly rewarding. So do not be discouraged. Progress, not perfection – is the key! If You Fall Off The Wagon, Stop! Identify the foods that caused you to stumble. What happened? What caused you to reach for the wrong food and put it in your mouth? Write about it in the journal where you wrote your food inventory. You can be certain that whichever food you ate is likely there in the 'banned' list, right? It isn't the end of the world.. .This process is, in many ways, like working out. If you are out of shape, at first you probably won't be able to life much weight. But, if you are persistent and keep at it, little by little you will get better at it. Losing weight and learning to eat is like mastering any task. If you have been overweight for a long time, you have to also confront the emotional addiction that we have to many of these foods. The more you practice the cleansing diet, the more all of this will fade and the closer you will get to your ultimate goal and freedom. I can guarantee you that this is the truth because such was the case with me. So don't ever give up. Keep moving forward.

Chapter 10
A Word From Rocky Balboa

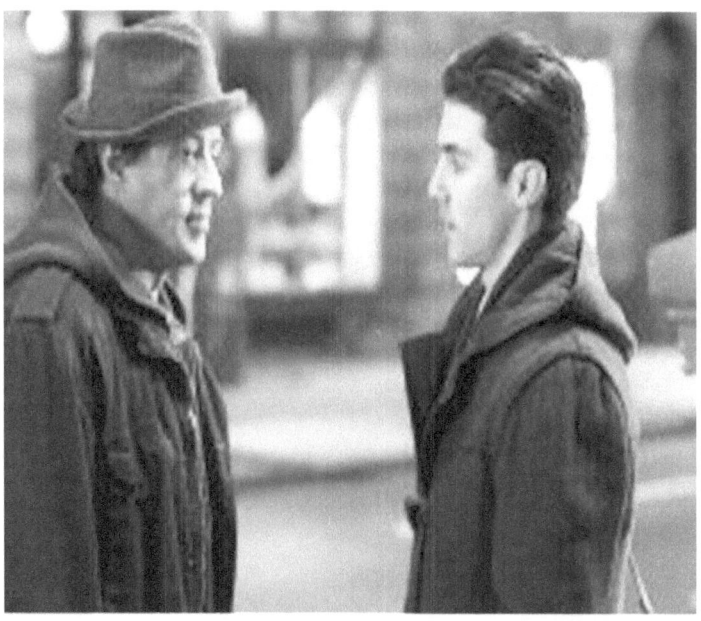

There is a quote from the 2006 movie Rocky Balboa that I like to remind myself of. Rocky tells his son:

"Let me tell you something you already know. The world ain't all sunshine and rainbows. It's a very mean and nasty place, and I don't care how tough you are, it will beat you to your knees and keep you there permanently if you let it. You, me, or nobody is gonna hit as hard as life. But it ain't about how hard you hit. It's about how hard you can get hit and keep moving forward; how much you can take and keep moving forward. That's how winning is done! Now, if you know what you're worth, then go out and get what you're worth. But you gotta be willing to take the hits, and not pointing fingers saying you ain't where you wanna be because of him, or her, or anybody. Cowards do that and that ain't you. You're better than that!

Chapter 11
The 5 D's

In closing, let me share with you the five key steps (*which I call the Five D's*) which helped me to hang on, even when the symptoms and hunger were at their worst. Take your time and put these to practice thoroughly as I know that they will help you a lot.

***DECIDE** that you are through with the old way of things. Look at the goals that you have related to your health, weight and eating. Resolve in your heart-of-hearts that you ARE going to follow through - no matter what. Draw an imaginary line that ends your old way of eating and relating to food, health and wellness, and become totally willing in your inner self to take the action to change **PERMANENTLY** – one day at a time.

***DEFINE** the type of life that you want to have as a result of your new healthy lifestyle. Look at the new avenues, activities and relationships you want to engage in as you move forward. So, as of now, (*if you* *haven't done so already*) mark that calendar and decide when you intend to start with this cleansing diet. If you have truly defined the type of life that you want for yourself, then moving forward with your weight loss and health-improvement goals is an absolute must. And I'm not talking about tomorrow, next week or next month. I am talking about **RIGHT HERE AND RIGHT NOW!.**

*DECLARE** to your close friends and family that you are through with being overweight and toxic and that you will be implementing some changes during the next months to lose weight and get. Tell them that you will **NO LONGER** be indulging in junk food and that you do not wish for it to be offered.

The purpose of this step is to give you some immediate accountability with persons that know you. It is not the same to sneak a pizza when nobody knows what you are doing! You do not, however, have to disclose your plans to everyone. Disclose it only to immediate family members, of course... people that you trust and you know will not judge or try to put banana peels in your path. You may not realize it, but there are people who will resent that you are taking action to get a hold of your life and health. Be aware and don't let them bring you down!

*DESIGNATE** a specific person that you trust and tell him or her specifically what you intend to do and why. Ask this person for support during the process and stay accountable to him or her on a regular basis. Visit **FitnessThroughFasting.com** and go to the forums where you can give and receive lots of support and motivation.

There are tons of online forums dedicated to weight loss. Find one that you feel comfortable in and make it a point to get involved with the community.

That alone will help you in more ways that you can imagine. In short, this step is designed so that you can determine which person in your close circle would best be suited to support you in the coming nine-months.

*DEVELOP** a strong journal where you can put in writing the reasons why it is important **FOR YOU** to reach your weight loss goals. Some examples can be; *weight loss, better health, healing from specific illnesses, more energy and vitality, mental clarity, dropping clothing sizes to a particular size, participating in a certain sport, getting married, dating, wearing a bathing suit you always wanted to, having a flat stomach, getting into your high-school-days clothing etc...*

These are personal reasons and are crucial because they mean something **TO YOU**... not to your spouse, children or family... but TO YOU. Yes, our loved ones are an immense source of motivation to get us going, but ultimately we have to do this **FOR OURSELVES!**

I cannot stress enough the importance of keeping a journal. In it, you can write the **dreams and goals that are closest to your he**art. You can write exactly what you want to get out of your weight loss efforts.

And those dreams and goals are the powerhouse of your spirit and mind. Each time you find yourself weak and wanting to give in, you can pick up the journal and read what you have written.

During those moments of weakness, **REMEMBER** the huge payoff in health and weight loss that you will receive. Learn that "a *life worth living is a life worth recording.*"

See you in the next volume! :-)

ROBERT DAVE JOHNSTON

Grab The Entire Collection:

Volume 1: The 'Permanent Weight Loss' Diet

Volume 2: The Intermittent Fasting Weight Loss Formula

Volume 3: How to Lose 30 Pounds (Or More) In 30 Days With Juice Fasting

Volume 4: Lose The Belly Fat Fast, And For Good!

Volume 5: Lose the Emotional Baggage: Transform Your Mind & Spirit With Fasting

Volume 6: How to Break a Fast (or Diet) and Keep The Weight Off

Volume 7: Compilation Volumes 1-6 -> Get All 5 For The Price Of 3!

Also by Robert Dave Johnston:

How To Lose Weight & Keep it Off By Transforming The Mind & Behaviors

Volume 1: How to Build a Rock-Solid Foundation That Supports Long-Term Weight Loss

Volume 2: How To Lose Weight & Keep it Off By Reprogramming The Subconscious Mind

Volume 3: How To Beat Diet Hunger and Junk Food Cravings

Volume 4: How to Escape the Diet "Time Trap" and Succeed in Weight Loss

Volume 5: How To Cheat On Your Diet (And Get Away With It)

Volume 6, Compilation: Get all 5 For The Price Of 3

Also By Robert Dave Johnston:

Detoxify Your Body, Lose Weight, Get Healthy & Transform Your Life

Volume 1- The 10-Day 'At Home' Colon Cleansing Formula

Volume 2- The 30-Day Kidney, Parasite & Liver Detox Weight Loss Method

Volume 3- Lose Weight Fast & Detoxify With Intermittent Fasting & At-Home Coffee Enemas

Volume 4 - Compilation: Get All 4 For The Price Of 2! Detoxify Your Body, Lose Weight, Get Healthy & Transform Your Life - Volumes 1-3

Don't forget to check the articles and growing health community at: FitnessThroughFasting.com